Meal Prep:

The Practical Guide to Preparing Quick, Delicious Meals for Weigh Loss, No Stress and Faster Fat Burning Results

The follow eBook is reproduced below with the goal of providing information that is as accurate and reliable as possible. Regardless, purchasing this eBook can be seen as consent to the fact that both the publisher and the author of this book are in no way experts on the topics discussed within and that any recommendations or suggestions that are made herein are for entertainment purposes only. Professionals should be consulted as needed prior to undertaking any of the action endorsed herein.

This declaration is deemed fair and valid by both the American Bar Association and the Committee of Publishers Association and is legally binding throughout the United States.

Furthermore, the transmission, duplication or reproduction of any of the following work including specific information will be considered an illegal act irrespective of if it is done electronically or in print. This extends to creating a secondary or tertiary copy of the work or a recorded copy and is only allowed with express written consent from the Publisher. All additional right reserved.

The information in the following pages is broadly considered to be a truthful and accurate account of facts and as such any inattention, use or misuse of the information in question by the reader will render any resulting actions solely under their purview. There are no scenarios in which the publisher or the original author of this work can be in any fashion deemed liable for any hardship or damages that may befall them after undertaking information described herein.

Additionally, the information in the following pages is intended only for informational purposes and should thus be thought of as universal. As befitting its nature, it is presented without assurance regarding its prolonged validity or interim quality. Trademarks that are mentioned are done without written consent and can in no way be considered an endorsement from the trademark holder.

Table of Contents

Introduction

Congratulations on downloading *Meal Prep: The Practical Guide to Preparing Quick Delicious Meals for Weight Loss, No Stress, And Faster Fat-Burning Results,* and thank you for doing so.

The following chapters will discuss techniques and recipes you can use to plan and prepare healthy meals ahead of time, make cooking easy and get control of your eating habits for weight loss.

Business is booming for startup companies that deliver a weekly box of pre-portioned ingredients. Even those who have advanced cooking skills may be held back from their fitness goals by a lack of time to prepare healthy lunches and well-balanced dinners.

You probably know a whole lot about healthy eating already, but maybe you're having trouble finding the time to cook wholesome food for yourself and your family. When you cook at home using whole ingredients, you'll be using your brain to put together well-balanced meals ahead of time. With a fridge stocked with meals and snacks that are ready-to-go, there's less of a chance that you'll fall prey to cravings or the urge to place a takeout order.

There are plenty of books on this subject on the market, thanks again for choosing this one! Every effort was made to ensure it is full of as much useful information as possible, please enjoy!

Chapter 1: Essential Meal Prepping Techniques

Schedule

One question you'll need to answer is how far in advance you'd like to cook. Will you prepare your meals for the next month, next week, or simply the next few days? Also ask yourself when you will make the time to do meal prep. Some people like to do two weekly shops, one on Sunday and one on Wednesday. If, on the other hand, you're ambitious enough to tackle an entire month, you'll want to consider bringing a buddy to pull an extra cart, or maybe splitting your shopping between two separate stores. If you're doing a big shop, plan to grab your fresh and frozen perishables last, to make sure they stay that way.

Also, look at your schedule for the week. Are there any days where you or members of your household will be out of town, or eating out? Before you plan for any week, make sure to ask yourself if there's any meal or day that you don't need to cook for.

And make sure you plan out *every* meal and snack that you need. This reduces stress and is one of the keys to meal prep for weight loss.

Portioning

If you want to lose weight, consider an online tool to calculate your daily calorie needs. Most of these tools will also allow you to determine your calorie requirements to reach your goal weight within a chosen amount of time.

Another consideration is how many people you are feeding in your household, and how far ahead you are cooking. This will decide how many meals you need to prepare at once. You may choose to double or triple the recipes in this book. Keep in mind that you may need more time to cook multiple batches one after another, or you may need more equipment.

Cook from scratch fast

Cutting up vegetables before the week starts gets them ready to add to your recipes. Often, the few extra steps it takes to put together a fresh meal are enough to get us off track. After a long day, the lineup of repetitive tasks required to prepare a salad can be a serious disincentive to eating healthy. When you get home late on Thursday night, your tomatoes and onions will be ready for your garden salad, and you'll be that much less likely to order up expensive and calorie-laden take-out. Your prepped-ahead veggies are good for more than just salad. They are equally useful for throwing together a colorful stir-fry, assembling a tasty pasta dish or bagging up healthy snacks for your family with items such as pepper slices or carrot sticks. Be sure to cook your protein ahead of time as well for ease of use. This book includes a number of recipes for meat that you can roast in the oven or in the slow cooker while you chop your vegetables for the week.

In fact, pasta and stir-fry deserve special mention here as two great go-to weeknight meals. Quickly assembled and endlessly modifiable, if you make them weekly standards, you'll knock out your meal planning for dinner two nights a week. Plan for a double batch, and you can have leftovers for dinner the next day.

One of the best things about these two dishes is that it's simple to adjust them to your dietary needs. Whole grain pasta is great, and you can also used spiralized veggies such as carrots or zucchini in place of traditional noodles. Stir fry can be served over brown rice, wild rice, cauliflower rice, or another grain such as quinoa or farro.

When you go to throw together a pasta dish, you can begin with a variety of sauces, such as tomato, pesto, or simple oil-and-garlic. Ramp up the nutritional value with some veggie add-ins. Sautee or mix in your pre-roasted asparagus, squash, mushrooms, onions, eggplant, cauliflower, or peppers. Zucchini, green peppers and onions is a trio that goes particularly well together.

Salads are another great go-to meal, both for dinner and lunch. Some people like to get inspiration for salads from restaurants. Unlike other dishes, salads have most of their ingredients (apart from the dressing) listed right there on the menu. Salads are also easy to improvise. Just toss some greens with a variety of your pre-chopped vegetables and a homemade dressing using one of your spice blends mixed with plain oil and vinegar, pureed avocado, or, most low-calorie of all, a squeeze of lemon. Make your salad a full meal by including some whole-wheat bread, or topping it with a whole grain, starchy vegetable or beans. As far as greens go, whatever you prefer is fine, but consider that any lettuce contains a negligible amount of vitamins. You'll get a more complete package by using spinach or kale.

Chop smart

When you're using whole, fresh vegetables, there's an easy way and a hard way to cut them up. Here's a trick that works equally well for bell peppers, apples, pears, broccoli, and cauliflower: holding the produce upright, slice down around the core, and rotate as you go. So, for example, with a round fruit or bell pepper, you will end up with four quarters of the fruit, the first with a circular imprint, the middle two will each be a third smaller, and the final cut will leave you with a more narrow strip. The end result is a pile of flesh with the core removed. You can then chop your pieces into smaller wedges or florets as needed. This trick also works for cabbage, chili peppers and corn.

Use your equipment

Slow cooker: Some observant users of slow cookers have remarked that it's impossible to set it, forget it, and come back to a perfectly cooked meal. This is because, these days, we're gone too long during the day. The optimal cooking time for many slow cooker recipes is around 6-7 hours, yet most shifts are at least eight hours, and that doesn't account for overtime work and time spent commuting. Whether or not that slow cooker chili is too sloppy depends on personal taste. But if you're faced with this problem, one way around is to use the slow cooker on days when you're sticking around home base.

Food processor: Although food processors have been around for a while, it's worth highlighting their everlasting usefulness. They're number one for creating tasty pesto, salsas, spice pastes and sauces. Several of their attachments are especially well-suited for meal prep. The grating feature is excellent for preparing vegetables for slaws, veggie burgers and salads. Try grinding a cup of nuts to keep on hand as a salad topping.

Chapter 2: Ingredients

- Healthy carbs: potatoes, sweet potatoes, rice, quinoa, farrow, bulgur, lentils, whole wheat pasta

- Lean proteins: beef, chicken, turkey, salmon, tuna, meatballs, eggs, pork loin or chops

- Green vegetables: kale, broccoli, spinach, green beans

- Vegetables for roasting: pumpkin, zucchini, broccoli, cauliflower, green beans, carrots, pumpkin

- Beans: full of protein and fiber and low in fat, beans, dried peas and lentils are all great foundations for a main course or a side dish.

The food groups above are the building blocks for your meal plans. This is meal prep at its simplest. Each ingredient can be seasoned and cooked simply on its own. Combine three of these basic dishes together, and you have yourself an easy meal.

If you're looking for more inspiration, the recipes in this book for breakfast and dinner are elements that each offer multiple possibilities for combination. Each of the lunch recipes stands on its own with around 400-500 calories and at least 7 grams of protein.

Chapter 3: Foods to Avoid

Here is a list of foods that don't store well:

1. Fish doesn't keep very long in the refrigerator. if you buy fresh fish, it should be your top priority to cook or freeze it right away.

2. Deep fried food doesn't do well in the freezer or the fridge.

3. Raw "salad" vegetables don't freeze well. This includes lettuce, radishes, tomatoes and onions.

4. Tomatoes gain a mealy texture when refrigerated, however, once roasted, they freeze beautifully.

5. Dairy, including cheese, sour cream, milk, does not freeze well. Hard cheese loses its texture but can still be used in recipes, however, you probably don't want to serve it on its own. Soft cheeses, sour cream, and milk tend to separate when frozen, so you may want to stir them before use.

6. Soup needs special treatment before it's frozen. Cooked potatoes, grains and noodles in soup all don't freeze well. It's best to undercook your noodles and grains if you're going to freeze the soup. Add the potatoes in as a raw ingredient directly before freezing. That way, these ingredients will cook as you reheat the soup.

When frozen, cooked egg whites gain a rubbery texture that is unpleasant to many people.

Chapter 4: Food Storage Advice

There are many opinions on how long it's ok to keep food. Some people rely on the smell test, and some people look for signs of mold. The FDA has released "short and safe" recommendations for food storage, included below:

FOOD	HOME REFRIGERATION PERIOD	FREEZER
Cooked Meat, Poultry and Fish Leftovers		
Pieces and cooked casseroles	3-4 days	2-3 months
Gravy and broth, patties and nuggets	3-4 days	2-3 months
Soups and stews	3-4 days	2-3 months
Fresh Fish and Shellfish	1-2 days	2-3 months
Fresh Meat		
Steaks, chops, roasts	3-5 days	2-3 months
Chicken, sausage, ground meat, stew meat	1-2 days	2-3 months
Bacon, ham, smoked sausage	7 days	1-2 months
Eggs		
Fresh eggs, in shell	3-5 weeks	Don't freeze
Hard-cooked eggs	1 week	Don't freeze

Freezer tips

When freezing foods, follow the food storage guidelines above. Never thaw meat and refreeze it. The second most important rule when it comes to freezing is to acquire the right packaging. You will need freezer bags, containers with airtight lids, heavy aluminum foil, plastic wrap, and freezer bags. If you are trying to limit your use of plastic, good for you! You can freeze things in glass jars, just leave head room for the food to expand when freezing. If you are freezing food in smaller portions, you can freeze it in sandwich bags, placing the smaller bags within a larger, well-labeled freezer bag.

Let food cool before you put it away, otherwise it may lower the temperature of your entire fridge or freezer, and all the other foods in there.

Casseroles, like the enchiladas in this book, should be put in the freezer without cooking beforehand.

Label everything: always, always, always label your freezer food. Include the name of the dish, the date it was frozen, and any important instructions you'll want to remember. If there's a layer of plastic wrap hidden under a layer of foil, you will probably want to give yourself a gentle reminder to take off the plastic before you put it in the oven!

Chapter 5: Meal Prep Hacks

Flavor secrets

Frozen flavor bombs: The ice cube tray is your secret weapon for freezing tender herbs, stock, or leftover tomato paste. For herbs, remove most of the stems, then blanch in boiling water for about a minute, or until bright green. Allow the herbs to cool before portioning into the tray. Get creative and make your own flavor bombs. Add in some minced ginger and grated garlic before you freeze for a great addition to Indian, Thai, and Chinese dishes.

Spice mixes: how many steps can you remove if you're not measuring 10 individual spices for your soup, meats, or roasted vegetables? Buy spice mixes like curry powder, za'atar, seasoning salt, spice rubs or five-spice powder, or create your own.

Quality over quantity: Cheese is a delicious addition to any meal, but it adds unwanted calories and fat. Keep the flavor of cheese and lose the drawbacks by looking for the best quality, strongest variety at the store. You'll find that you're more satisfied with a smaller amount.

Make it a party

Meal prep doesn't have to be a solo affair. Invite a friend over and double your recipes and you'll both have food for the week. Choose your recipes beforehand to make sure you're cooking food you both like. If you're cooking for your family, include your partner or children. Cooking with kids teaches them a valuable skill and will have the added benefit of familiarizing them with new ingredients, which can make them more likely to eat their vegetables! Many food preparation activities are child-friendly, or can be made child-friendly. For example, peeling vegetables and forming meatballs are fun and easy tasks. Consider setting up a chopping station for your younger children, and give them a butter knife for cutting soft vegetables like potatoes and zucchini, or safety scissors for snipping herbs.

Another idea to make meal prep a social event is to have a food exchange. Send your friends and family this eBook, and set a date for your frozen potluck. Perhaps you might also email the group in advance and ask them what their favorite meals are, to make sure the individual recipes have wide appeal. You might also choose a theme, like a winter soup or casserole exchange. Everyone should prepare a family-sized portion of the chosen recipe in a quantity equaling the size of the group.

Finally, you can use meal prep to do good. Maybe you know someone with a new baby, or who has lost a loved one, or just someone going through a tough time. Bring them an entrée or two, and you'll know you did your part to help.

Keep it visible

To make sure that all the time and money you've put into shopping and preparing your food doesn't go to waste, it helps to catalogue what's in your kitchen. Index both your fridge and your freezer, and, optimally, your pantry as well. Keep a list posted on the fridge door, hanging on the wall, or in a notebook, inventorying the food you've so lovingly prepared.

Another tip is to keep your ingredients out when you get back from the store. This tip is for the procrastinators in particular. If you have a couple of days or hours in between your shop and prep time, seeing your cans of beans and bag of rice on the counter is a visual reminder and motivator for your meal prep. Having some of your ingredients out helps remove one small step from the task of cooking, and gets you a little closer to starting your task.

Lastly, organize your kitchen to make your most-used items at the forefront. Keep jars of beans, rice and other grains on the counter, if you have space. It's likely that you will use garlic, ginger and onions often, so place them in a bowl where you'll have easy access to them. Be sure to store spices in a manner that allows you to quickly find what you need. Use a spice rack, or a lazy Susan.

Chapter 6: Breakfast

Smoothie freezer packs

Smoothies are a great way to start the day, but who has the time to portion out all the ingredients during the morning rush? Additionally, some smoothies incorporate fresh ingredients that might go bad before you use them. Save yourself some time by portioning out the ingredients ahead of time. Here are the general directions for the recipes in this category.

1. *Place ingredients in individual sandwich bags.*

2. *Put smaller bags in a large gallon freezer bag.*

3. *To make a smoothie, dump ingredients into a blender and add 1 cup water to loosen it up. The nutrition facts for this recipe use water, but you can also use dairy, soy, almond, coconut or rice milk.*

Enjoy a smoothie on its own, or as part of a balanced breakfast using the egg muffins or breakfast burrito. This would also make a great after-work or after-school treat.

Purple smoothie

Ingredients
1 frozen banana
1 orange, peeled
1 cup organic frozen mixed berries
6oz Vanilla Greek Yogurt

Nutrition Facts Serves: 1
Calories 330Calories From Fat 45, Total Fat 5g, Saturated Fat 1g, Trans Fat 0g, Cholesterol 20mg 7%, Sodium 85mg, Potassium 30%, Total Carbohydrates 65g%, Dietary Fiber 13g, Sugars 23g, Protein 8g, Vitamin A 15%, Vitamin C 240%, Calcium 35%, Iron10%

Power green smoothie with kiwi

Ingredients
1/2 avocado
1 frozen banana sliced
2 kiwis peeled and chopped
1/2 cup vanilla yogurt
1/2 cup kale very finely chopped

Nutrition Facts Serves: 1
Calories 430, Calories From Fat 180, Total Fat 20g, Saturated Fat 1g, Trans Fat 0g, Cholesterol 1 mg, Sodium 75mg, Potassium 46%, Total Carbohydrates 65g, Dietary Fiber 15g, Sugars 34g, Protein 9g, Vitamin A 70%, Vitamin C 290%, Calcium 25%

Simple and light green smoothie

Ingredients
1 frozen banana
1 handfuls baby spinach
3/4 cup orange juice

Nutrition Facts Serves: 1
Calories 140, Total Fat 0g, Cholesterol 0 mg, Trans Fat 0 g, Saturated Fat 0 g, Sodium 10mg, Potassium 17%, Total Carbohydrates 33g, Sugars 21g, Vitamin C 120%, Calcium4%, Dietary Fiber 3 g, Protein 2, Vitamin A 20 %

Minty mango and raspberry smoothie

Ingredients
10 spearmint leaves, rinsed
1/2 lime juiced
1 pinch sea salt
1 1/2 cups ice cubes
1 cup fresh raspberries
1 large mango, peeled and diced

Nutrition Facts Serves: 1
Calories 170, Total Fat 0g, Saturated Fat 0g, Trans Fat 0g, Cholesterol 0 mg, Sodium 110mg, Potassium 17%, Total Carbohydrates 45g, Dietary Fiber 9g, Sugars 32g, Vitamin A 70%, Vitamin C 130%, Calcium 15%, Iron 35%, Protein 4 g

Veggie egg muffins

These muffins are full of protein, and easy to reheat in the microwave. Just allow one minute per muffin, depending on the strength of your microwave. Feel free to substitute the cheese of your choice, and remember that a stronger cheese is more flavorful and satisfying.

Prep time: 20 minutes
Cook time: 30 minutes
Total time: 50 minutes

Ingredients
1 small onion, diced
4 medium mushrooms, sliced
2 tsp. powdered garlic
1 tsp. salt
1/4 cups provolone cheese, shredded
8 eggs
1/4 cup milk
2 cups Broccoli, cut or torn into small florets
1 cup chopped bell pepper

Sweet potato breakfast burrito

This burrito tastes better than any drive-thru breakfast sandwich, and you can prepare a whole batch in around half an hour. Reheat one burrito in about two minutes. It's fast food, and it has less than 300 calories per serving.

Prep time: 25 minutes
Cook time: 10 minutes
Total time: 35 minutes

Ingredients
4 tsp. olive oil
2 oz. shredded cheddar cheese
4 cups packed baby spinach, roughly chopped
2 small sweet potatoes, peeled and diced
2 small yellow onions, chopped
1 1/2 cup frozen, sliced tricolor bell peppers, thawed
8 9- or 10-inch whole wheat or gluten-free tortillas
2 tsp. chile powder
4 large eggs, beaten
4 large egg whites, beaten

Instructions

1. In a large skillet, heat the oil on medium heat. Sauté potato, onion and bell peppers for approximately 7 minutes. Toss in chili powder and spinach and sauté for another 2 minutes.

2. Turn heat up to medium high. Mix in eggs and egg whites. Cook for 3 minutes, continuing to stir, until eggs are cooked completely and not runny. Remove from heat and cool for 10 minutes.

3. Cut 8 16-inch pieces of aluminum foil. Place 1 tortilla on top of each piece. Put an equal portion of the egg mixture in the middle of each tortilla. Sprinkle cheese on top. Fold two sides in first, and then roll forward from the top of the burrito. Make sure the foil is wrapped tightly around the burrito, but not inside the roll, if you will be microwaving it to reheat.

4. Place burritos into a large plastic bag in the fridge. There are two ways to reheat. You can either bake the burrito on a cookie sheet in a 400 degree oven for 35 minutes, or cook in the microwave for 2 minutes. Transfer the burrito to a paper bag with a pair of tongs, and you can bring it with you on the run.

Nutrition Facts Serving size: 1 burrito

Calories: 255, Total Fat: 10 g, Sat. Fat: 3 g, Monounsaturated Fat: 5 g, Polyunsaturated Fat: 2 g, Carbs: 38 g, Fiber: 15.5 g, Sugars: 7 g, Protein: 17 g, Sodium: 465 mg, Cholesterol: 100 mg

Equipment

Ingredients
1 muffin tin

Instructions
1. Ensure your oven is heated to 350 degrees.
2. Grease the muffin pan, and fill with vegetables.
3. In a mixing bowl combine the eggs, garlic powder & salt.
4. Fill each cup 3/4 of the way with the egg mixture then top with a pinch of cheese.
5. Bake for about 25 to 30 minutes or until puffy and golden brown.

Nutrition Facts Serves: 8
Calories 130, Calories From Fat 65, Total Fat 7g, Saturated Fat 2.5g, Trans Fat 0g, Cholesterol 245mg, Sodium 315mg, Potassium 8.5%, Total Carbohydrates 6.5g, Dietary Fiber 1.5g, Sugars 3g, Protein 10.5g, Vitamin A 22.5%, Vitamin C 85%, Calcium 10%, Iron 10%

Chapter 7: Lunch

Black bean and red pepper quinoa salad

This is a filling salad that keeps well. It's under five hundred calories, but has a good deal of olive oil. Cut down on the calories by reducing some of the oil.

Prep time: 10 minutes
Cook time: 15 minutes
Time total: 25 minutes

Ingredients
Salad:
3/4 cup quinoa
1 1/2 cups water
1 pinch salt
1/3 cup thinly sliced green onion
1 red bell pepper, chopped into small dice
1/2 cup chopped cilantro
1 can black beans drained, rinsed

Dressing:
2 T. lime juice
1 tsp. seasoning salt of your choice
black pepper to taste
1 tsp. ground cumin
1/4 cup extra-virgin olive oil
1/2 tsp. paprika or other chili powder

Instructions

1. Rinse the quinoa in a fine-mesh strainer. Add quinoa, water, and salt. Bring to a boil, then simmer covered for 15 minutes, or until water is absorbed. Fluff up quinoa with a fork and let cool while you prepare the rest of the salad.

2. Drain the beans into a colander in the sink and rinse with cold water, until all the foam is gone. Drain beans until they are very dry (or pat with paper towels to speed it up.)

3. Dice the bell pepper finely. Slice the green onions thinly and wash, dry, and chop the cilantro.

4. Once the quinoa has cooled, combine it in a bowl with the black beans, diced red bell pepper, and sliced green onion. Portion it out into 8 containers and sprinkle some chopped cilantro on top. You can mix in the dressing right away or keep the dressing on the side and add in a little before eating. This meal will remain good for 3 days as long as it is refrigerated.

Nutrition Facts Servings: 4, Calories: 450, Calories From Fat: 150, Total Fat: 16g, Saturated Fat: 2g,Trans Fat: 0g, Cholesterol: 0mg, Sodium: 300mg, Potassium: 1140mg, Total Carbohydrates: 59g, Dietary Fiber: 12g, Sugars: 3g, Protein: 18g

Asparagus and farro salad

Farro is nutritionally very similar to quinoa, but has a delicious taste all of its own that some compare to rice. Make sure to get perlato, otherwise you will need to look up directions to cook other varieties of farro. Perlato is the quick-cooking variety.

Prep time: 20 minutes
Cook time: 30 minutes
Total time: 50 minutes

Ingredients:
1 cup perlato Farro
1 cup asparagus, sliced small
3 tsp. olive oil
1 tsp. lemon juice
2/3 cups green onions, sliced
1/2 cups parsley, chopped
1 diced red pepper

Dressing:
1/3 cups capers, juice included
3 T chopped sun-dried tomatoes
2 T parsley, chopped
1/3 cups vinegar (red wine)
1/3 cups olive oil
2 tsp. lemon juice
1 tsp. Dijon

Equipment:
Food processor or blender

Instructions:

1. Add the farro to a skillet before placing the skillet on the stove on top of a high/medium heat until it begins to brown. You will then want to turn off the heat before adding in 1 ¾ cups boiling water to the skillet, as well as a pinch of salt. Turn the burner to low and let it cook for 20 minutes. Add a small amount of water if necessary.) Drain excess water.

2. As the farro cooks, you will want to add the parsley, tomatoes and capers to a food processor and process well. Add the pureed results into a bowl before adding in the red wine vinegar, Dijon and lemon juice before adding in the olive oil and whisking well.

3. After the farro has cooled, add it to a separate bowl and add ¼ cups of the previous bowl into this one.

4. Add 2 tsp. olive oil olive oil in a heavy pan, and sauté asparagus slices for 5 minutes. Add in the remainder of the lemon juice and add the results to the bowl of farro

5. Dice red pepper, then add 1 tsp. of olive oil to the pan and sauté red pepper about 1 minutes. Add red pepper to the bowl with the farro mixture.

6. Add the chopped parsley and sliced green onions together in a bowl and mix well. Add dressing to your liking or keep on the side to add before serving. This will keep for 3 days in the fridge.

Nutrition Facts Serves: 4

Calories 460, Calories From Fat 280, Total Fat: 31g, Saturated Fat 4g;,Trans Fat 0g, Cholesterol 0mg, Sodium 560mg, Total Carbohydrates 42g, Dietary Fiber 8g, Sugars 3g, Protein 7g, Potassium 10%, Vitamin A 40%, Vitamin C 90%, Calcium 6%, Iron 25%

Black bean and chorizo stew

This is a simple black bean stew that gets a boost from smoky chorizo. Like Italian sausage, chorizo can be either sweet or spicy, so make sure you pick up your favorite kind.

Prep time: 15 minutes
Cook time: 75 minutes
Total time: 1 hour 30 minutes

Ingredients

2 T olive oil
1 large white onion, diced
7 cups cooked black beans (from 4 cans or 1 pound dried beans), drained
1 (28-oz.) can diced plum tomatoes
12 oz. chorizo
¼ cup chopped cilantro stems, leaves reserved for serving
2 tsp. kosher salt, more as needed
Sliced scallion, for serving
Lime wedges, for serving
Diced avocado, for serving

Instructions

1. Place the oil in a heavy pot before placing the pot on the stove on top of a burner set to a medium heat. Add onion and cook, stirring occasionally, until softened, 5 to 10 minutes. Add in chorizo and the cilantro stems and cook an additional 5 minutes over high heat.
2. Stir in beans, tomatoes and their juices, and the water. Let the results boil, before reducing to medium.
3. Cover the pot partially and simmer until tomatoes fall apart, between 1 hour and 1 hour 15 minutes. Top with avocado, scallion, cilantro leaves and lime wedges to serve.

4. Portion into plastic containers or freezer bags. This recipe keeps in the fridge for 3-4 days and in the freezer for 2-3 months.

<u>Nutrition Facts</u> Serves: 6

431 calories; 26 grams fat; 8 grams saturated fat; 13 grams monounsaturated fat; 2 grams polyunsaturated fat; 26 grams carbohydrates; 8 grams dietary fiber; 4 grams sugars; 21 grams protein; 49 milligrams cholesterol; 1344 milligrams sodium

Chicken quesadilla and avocado salsa

Quesadillas are a great alternative to sandwiches for lunchtime, and they seem to hold up a little better in the lunch bag also. The avocado sauce in this recipe keeps surprisingly well in the freezer or fridge. If refrigerating the sauce, squeeze half of a lime over the top. This will keep your sauce green and fresh!

Prep time: 25 minutes
Cook time: 20 minutes
Total time: 45 minutes

Ingredients
Quesadillas
4 gluten-free tortillas
1 cup shredded Monterey Jack cheese
2 cups baby spinach leaves lightly packed
4 oz. diced green chills
8 oz. cooked chicken breast (shredded or cut into cubes)

Avocado Sauce
1 avocado, smashed
1 or 2 jalapeño peppers, seeded, halved
2 T lime juice
2 T olive oil
2 T Parmesan cheese, optional
1 clove garlic
1/2 tsp. salt
1 cup cilantro

Equipment
Blender or food processor

Instructions

1. Add all avocado sauce ingredients to a blender or food processor and blend until smooth.
2. Place a skillet on top of the stove over a burner set to a medium heat before adding in a tortilla, 1 T green chilies, ¼ cups of cheese, ½ cup spinach and ¼ of the total chicken.
3. Fold the results in half and let it cook for 2 minutes per side, repeat until all the ingredients have been used.
4. Slice up the quesadillas and serve with the avocado sauce. They can be wrapped in foil and refrigerated for 3-4 days or frozen for 2-3 months. Reheat in a toaster oven for best results

Nutrition facts: Serves: 4

Calories: 451, Total Fat: 25 g, Sat. Fat: 7 g, Polyunsaturated Fat: 3 g, Carbs: 31 g, Fiber: 8.5 g, Sugars: 1 g, Protein: 26 g, Sodium: 599 mg, Cholesterol: 58 mg, Monounsaturated Fat: 12 g

Turkey and white bean chili

White chili is a great alternative to the usual tomato sauce and ground beef version. The lime wedges are a great accompaniment, and contribute to a lighter, brighter taste.

Prep time: 15 minutes
Cook time: 1 hour 10 minutes
Total time: 1 hour 25 minutes

Ingredients
1 T canola oil
2 cups diced yellow onion
1 tsp. dried oregano
3 (15.8 oz.) cans Great Northern beans
2 T fresh lime juice
4 cups fat-free, low sodium chicken broth
3 cups chopped cooked turkey*
1/2 cup diced seeded plum tomato (about 1)
1/3 cup chopped cilantro
1 T minced garlic
1 1/2 tsp. cumin, ground
8 lime wedges (optional)
1/2 tsp. salt
Ground black pepper, to taste
1 1/2 T chili powder
*See next recipe for Roast Turkey Breast

Equipment
Dutch oven or heavy-bottomed pan
Blender or food processor

Instructions

1. Place a pan with a heavy bottom on top of the stove over a burner set to a high/medium heat. Add onion and sauté for 10 minutes or until soft and golden. Add the chili powder, garlic, and cumin and stir for 2 minutes. Add oregano and beans, and cook for a brief 30 seconds. Let the broth simmer and cook for 20 minutes.

2. Place 2 cups of bean mixture in a blender or food processor, and blend until smooth. Return the pureed mixture to the Dutch oven. Add turkey, and cook 5 minutes or until thoroughly heated through. Remove pan from heat. Add diced tomato, chopped cilantro, lime juice, salt, and pepper to finish and stir well. Serve with lime wedges, if you like.

Nutrition Facts Serves: 12

Calories 286, Calories from fat 19 %, Fat 6 g, Saturated fat 1.2 g, Monounsaturated fat 2.1 g, Polyunsaturated fat 1.6 g, Protein 32.4 g, Carbohydrate 24.3 g, Fiber 5.5 g, Cholesterol 85 mg, Iron 4.8 mg, Sodium 435 mg, Calcium 105 mg

Roast turkey breast

This roast turkey would also go well in a sandwich and can stand on its own as a main dish. Make this recipe your own by using your favorite seasoning blend instead of the spices mentioned here.

Prep time: 5 minutes
Cook time: 1 hour 30 minutes
Total time: 1 hour 35 minutes

Ingredients
1 tsp. dry onion, minced
½ tsp. powdered garlic
2 T extra virgin olive oil
2 lb. turkey breast, boneless
½ tsp. fresh basil
½ tsp. parsley, chopped
½ tsp. black pepper
1 tsp. paprika, smoked
1 tsp. seasoning salt

Equipment
Roasting pan

Instructions
1. Let the turkey thaw before ensuring your oven is heated to 350 degrees Fahrenheit.
2. In a small bowl, combine all of the seasonings thoroughly.
3. Rub turkey first with the olive oil and then the spice mixture.
4. Place 3 aluminum balls at the bottom of the baking pan before adding in the turkey breast.
5. Place the turkey in the oven and let it bake for 90 minutes until the internal temperature is at least 165 degrees Fahrenheit.
6. After taking the turkey out of the oven, cover using tinfoil and let it sit for 20 minutes prior to slicing.

Nutrition Facts Serves: approximately 8 (serving size 4 oz.) Calories 160, Sodium 390 mg, Fat 7 g, Saturated fat 2 g, Protein 21 g, Cholesterol 65 mg

Chapter 8: Dinner

No noodle lasagna

Consider using the technique for roasted spaghetti squash to create a substitute for noodles in any pasta dish.

Prep time: 10 minutes
Cook time: 1 hour 35 minutes
Total time: 1 hour 45 minutes

Ingredients:
1 large ripe spaghetti squash
salt and fresh pepper
2 cups marinara sauce
1 cup part skim ricotta
8 tsp. parmesan cheese
6 oz. shredded part skim mozzarella

Equipment:
Disposable foil 5x7 inch baking pans

Instructions:
*See next recipe for roasted spaghetti squash.
1. Preheat oven to 375 degrees Fahrenheit.
2. Cut the squash in half, and scoop out all the seeds and fibers with a spoon.
3. Place on a baking sheet, with the cut side up, and season with the salt and pepper.
4. Bake at 375 degrees Fahrenheit about an hour or until the skin gives easily under pressure and the inside is tender. Remove from oven and let it cool for 10 minutes.
5. Use a fork to create "noodles" from the squash. It will fluff up into spaghetti-like strands.

6. Pour 1/4 cup quick marinara sauce on the bottom of four individual 5 x 7-inch pans. Top the sauce with 3/4 cup of the spaghetti squash and spread evenly. Add ¼ the total ricotta to each, top with mozzarella. Add mozzarella and bake for 10 minutes.

Nutrition Facts: Serves: 4, Calories 370, Calories From Fat 180, Total Fat 20g, Saturated Fat 10g, Trans Fat 0g, Cholesterol 55mg, Sodium 940mg, Potassium 18%, Total Carbohydrates 29g, Dietary Fiber 4g, Sugars 12g, Protein 21g, Vitamin A 30%, Vitamin C 8%, Calcium 45%, Iron 8%

Roasted Italian chicken with vegetables

Here is a great example of a meal prep recipe where you can deploy your pre-chopped vegetables for an easy weeknight meal.

Prep time: 20 minutes
Cook time: 25 minutes
Total time: 45 minutes

Ingredients:
2 sage leaves, chopped
½ T thyme, dried
1 ½ T rosemary
½ tsp. sugar
2 garlic cloves, chopped, smashed
2 red bell peppers
10 asparagus stalks, cut in half with their ends trimmed
2 T olive oil
Ground black pepper, as needed
Cooking spray
¼ cup + 1 T balsamic vinegar (divided)
5 oz. mushrooms, sliced
½ cups carrots, prepared in 3-inch chunks
1 red onion, chopped
1 tsp. kosher salt
8 chicken thighs, 4 oz.

Instructions:

1. Ensure your oven is heated to 425 degrees Fahrenheit.
2. Season the chicken using the pepper as well as the salt and grease a pair of baking sheets using the cooking spray
3. Using a large bowl, combine the sage, thyme, rosemary, sugar, garlic, red bell peppers, asparagus, balsamic vinegar, mushrooms, carrots, onions, and chicken together and mix well before adding the results to the baking sheet. Ensure the vegetables and the chicken are not touching.
4. Place the baking sheets into the oven and let everything cook for 20 minutes until the chicken reaches an internal temperature that is at least 16 degrees and the vegetables are appropriately steamed.

Nutrition Facts Serves: 6

Calories 210, Calories From Fat 100, Total Fat 11g, Saturated Fat 15g, Trans Fat 0g, Cholesterol 0mg, Sodium 190mg, Potassium 690mg, Total Carbohydrates 23g, Dietary Fiber 6g, Sugars 13g, Protein 5g, Vitamin A 130%, Vitamin C 170%, Calcium 10%, Iron 20%

Slow cooker short ribs

Short ribs are a relatively cheap cut of meat that taste like a million dollars when you cook them with this recipe.

Prep time: 25 mins
Cook time: 8 hours
Total time: 8 hours 25 minutes

Ingredients
½ cup water
Salt and pepper
2 cubes beef stock
1 bay leaf
1 lb. baby carrots, peeled
14.5 oz. diced tomatoes, canned
½ cups mushrooms, sliced
1 T olive oil
3 thyme sprigs
3 garlic cloves, minced
1 onion, chopped
4 lb. short ribs, beef

Instructions

1. Add the oil to a skillet before placing in on the stove over a burner set to a high/medium heat. Season the ribs using pepper and salt as needed.
2. Add the ribs to the skillet and let them brown thoroughly before removing them from the skillet and placing them in a slow cooker.
3. Leave the pan where it is before turning the burner to a low/medium heat. Add the mushrooms, garlic and onion to the skillet and let them sauté for 3 minutes.
4. Clean out the pan before placing it back on the stove and adding in the cubes of beef stock as well as the thyme, carrots, bay and the full diced tomatoes can. Mix well before adding the results to the slow cooker.
5. Set the slow cooker to cook for 4 hours on high or 8 hours on low.
6. After the ribs have finished cooking, preheat your oven to 200 degrees before placing the ribs on a platter and covering in tinfoil to keep them warm.
7. Remove the juices from the slow cooker and place them in the skillet before placing the skillet on the stove on top of a burner set to a high/medium heat. Let the juices reduce for 5 minutes.
8. Cover ribs in sauce prior to serving with potatoes or rice. This recipe can be kept in the fridge for 3-4 days or in the freezer for 2-3 months.

Nutrition Facts Serves: 4

Calories 120, Calories From Fat 35, Total Fat 35g, Saturated Fat 5g, Trans Fat 0g, Cholesterol 0mg, Sodium 600mg, Potassium 18%, Total Carbohydrates 19, Dietary Fiber 6g, Sugars 10g, Protein 4g, Vitamin A330%, Vitamin C 35%, Calcium 8%, Iron 10%

Grilled chicken

Grilled chicken will give you a taste of summer any day of the year. High quality cast iron grill pans can be had for $25. Strips of these grilled chicken breasts will make any green salad a meal.

Prep time: 15 minutes
Cook time: 1 hour 15 minutes
Total time: 1 hour 30 minutes

Ingredients
Torn mint leaves, to taste
4 cloves garlic, peeled, crushed
2 T thyme chopped
2 T olive oil
2 lemons
Black pepper, to taste
1 ½ tsp. salt
4 chicken breasts, 6 oz. each, pounded to ½ inch thick

Equipment
Outdoor grill, George Forman grill, or cast-iron grill pan

Instructions
1. In a large bowl, place the chicken before seasoning with lemon juice and the zest of 1 lemon, garlic, thyme, pepper and salt and coat well. Let the chicken sit in the refrigerator for 1 hour.
2. Heat your grill before coating the chicken in olive oil and grilling each side for 4 minutes.
3. Top with mint leaves, olive oil and lemon juice prior to serving. They will keep in the fridge for 3-4 days or in the freezer for 2-3 months.

Nutrition Facts Serves: 4, Calories: 270, Sodium: 360 mg, Total Fat: 6 g, Potassium: 0 mg, Saturated: 2 g, Total Carbs: 0 g, Polyunsaturated: 1 g, Dietary Fiber: 0 g, Monounsaturated Fat: 3 g, Sugars: 0 g, Trans: 0 g, Protein: 32 g, Cholesterol: 90 mg

Turkey meatballs

Why not try these fast and easy turkey meatballs with some roasted spaghetti squash and tomato sauce?

Prep time: 5 minutes
Cook time: 15 minutes
Total time: 20 minutes

Ingredients
1 1/3 pounds ground turkey
2/3 cup dry breadcrumbs
1/8 cup coarsely shredded carrot
1/4 cup coarsely shredded zucchini
1/4 cup chopped fresh parsley
1/2 cup (2 oz.) finely shredded fresh parmesan cheese
1/3 cup finely chopped green onions
Salt, to taste
Pepper, to taste
1 egg
2 cloves garlic, crushed
Cooking spray

Instructions
1. Ensure your oven is heated to 400 degrees Fahrenheit.
2. In a large bowl, combine the garlic, egg, pepper, salt, green onions, parmesan cheese, parsley, zucchini, carrot, breadcrumbs and turkey and combine thoroughly.
3. Roll the mixture into 30 (1 1/2-inch) meatballs.
4. Add the results to a baking pan that has been coated thoroughly using cooking spray. Place the pan in the oven and let the meatballs cook for approximately 15 minutes.

Nutrition Facts Serves: 6 (5 meatballs) Calories 228, Calories from fat 70g, Fat 7.3 g, Saturated fat 3.1 g, Monounsaturated fat 1.8 g, Polyunsaturated fat 1.4 g, Protein 30.3 g, Carbohydrates 8.5 g, Fiber 0.8 g, Cholesterol 71 mg, Iron 2.5 mg, Sodium 399 mg, Calcium 166 mg

Root vegetable casserole

This is a tasty but relatively high fat dish that would do well prepped alongside some lean meat.

Prep time: 30 minutes
Cook time: 1 hour 30 minutes
Total time: 2 hours

Ingredients
Butter
1 cup heavy cream
6 T sour cream
1 cup whole milk
Ground black pepper, to taste
Sea salt, to taste
6 oz. cheddar cheese, grated
11 oz. celeriac, halved, peeled, sliced thin
13 oz. turnips, halved, peeled, sliced thin
1 ½ lbs. potatoes, halved, peeled, sliced thin
1 lb. rutabaga, halved, peeled, sliced thin

Equipment
8 by 12-inch baking dish

Instructions

1. Ensure your oven is heated to 400 degrees Fahrenheit. Butter an 8 by 12-inch baking dish.
2. In a mixing bowl, combine the slices of celeriac, turnip, potatoes and rutabaga together and mix well
3. Place a saucepan on the stove on top of a burner set to a low heat before adding in the milk, sour cream and regular cream and mix until combined. Remove the saucepan from the burner and season using pepper as well as salt and stir repeatedly.
4. Place half of the total amount of sliced root vegetables into a baking dish before seasoning using pepper and salt as needed as well as 1/3 of all of the cheese. Add a third of the total cream mixture to the top of the vegetables before adding in the rest of the vegetables and the rest of the cheese. Top with the rest of the cream.
5. Place the results in the oven and let them bake for 90 minutes until the top is well-browned. Allow to cool and portion out into containers or plastic bags. This recipe can be refrigerated for 3-4 days or frozen for 2-3 months.

Nutrition Facts Serves: 6 Calories 370, Calories From Fat 160, Total Fat 17g, Saturated Fat 11g, Trans Fat 0g, Cholesterol 55mg, Sodium 310mg, Potassium 33%, Total Carbohydrates 38g, Dietary Fiber 8g, Sugars 14g, Protein 15g, Vitamin A 10%, Vitamin C 120%, Calcium 45%, Iron 15%

Greek mixed roasted vegetables

You can serve these Greek vegetables with some brown rice for an amazing combination. You can also use dill in place of or in addition to the basil. This dish would be easy to prepare with some pre-chopped vegetables.

Prep time: 15 minutes
Cook time: 40 minutes
Total time: 1 hour

Ingredients
1 eggplant, peeled and diced 3/4-inch
Ground black pepper, to taste
Kosher sea salt, to taste
2 T extra virgin olive oil
2 cloves of garlic, minced
1 small onion, red, peeled, diced 1-inch
2 bell pepper red, yellow, diced, 1-inch

Dressing
1/4 cup olive oil
1/3 cup lemon juice, squeezed fresh
Ground black pepper, to taste
Kosher sea salt, to taste

Toppings
15 leaves of fresh basil
¾ lbs. feta, diced
4 scallions, minced

Instructions

1. Ensure your oven is heated to 425 degrees Fahrenheit.
2. One a sheet pan, combine the garlic, onion, yellow bell pepper, red bell pepper and eggplant before seasoning using the pepper, salt and olive oil.
3. Add the pan to the oven and let it cook for 40 minutes, using a spatula to flip everything after 20 minutes.
4. As the vegetables are cooking, combine the pepper, salt, olive oil and lemon juice together in a small bowl, add the results to the vegetables as soon as they come out of the oven.
5. Let the pan cool completely before adding in the basil, feta and scallions. Season prior to serving.

Nutrition Facts Serves: 4

Calories 95, Sodium 0mg, Total fat 9g, Potassium 0mg, Saturated fat 0g, Total Carbs 3g, Polyunsaturated fat 0g, Dietary Fiber 0g, Monounsaturated fat 0g, Sugars 0g, Trans fat 0g, Protein 1g, Cholesterol 0 mg

Autumn roasted green beans

Blistering the green beans elevates this fall vegetable dish. In addition to using it in your meal prep rotation, it may even be worthy of inclusion in your Thanksgiving menu.

Prep time: 15 minutes
Cook time: 30 minutes
Total time: 45 minutes

Ingredients
½ cups toasted walnuts
½ cups cranberries, dried
Ground black pepper, to taste
Kosher sea salt to taste
2 tsp. lemon juice
1 tsp. lemon zest
¼ tsp. sugar
2 T olive oil
4 garlic cloves, quartered and peeled
2 lbs. green beans, stems trimmed

Instructions
1. Preheat your oven to 350 degrees Fahrenheit and crack and smash the walnuts in to chunks.
2. Spread the walnuts onto a baking sheet and toast them for 10 minutes.
3. Increase the temperature on the oven to 450 degrees Fahrenheit.
4. Cover a baking sheet with a rim using aluminum foil.
5. In a mixing bowl, combine the sugar, pepper, salt and olive oil before coating the garlic and green beans thoroughly.
6. Place the beans onto a baking sheet and spread them out to ensure they cook well. Place the sheet into the oven and let

the beans bake for 15 minutes, before stirring with a spatula and roasting another 10 minutes.

7. Mix in the lemon juice, pepper and salt prior to serving.

Nutrition Facts Serves: 7, Calories 130, Total Fat 7g, Saturated Fat 1g, Sodium 230mg, Potassium 8%, Total Carbohydrates 16 g, Sugars 8 g, Protein 2 g, Vitamin A 15%, Calcium 6%, Iron 8%, Dietary Fiber 3 g, Vitamin C 25%

Roasted summer squash

This is a summery dish that would pair well with the recipe for slow cooker pulled pork. Use your favorite seasoned salt in place of the salt and pepper, if desired.

Prep time: 5 minutes
Cook time: 30 minutes
Total time: 35 minutes

Ingredients
3 zucchini
3 yellow squash
1 ½ T kosher salt
½ T black pepper
2 T extra-virgin olive oil

Instructions
1. Ensure your oven is heated to 400 degrees Fahrenheit
2. Peel vegetables and cut into ¼ inch thick slices.
3. Assemble vegetables on a baking sheet or pan and drizzle olive oil on top. Sprinkle with pepper and salt as needed
4. Bake at 400 degrees Fahrenheit for 30 minutes.

Nutrition Facts Serves: 6 Calories 80, Calories From Fat 40, Total Fat 4g, Saturated Fat 5g, Trans Fat 0g, Cholesterol 0mg, Sodium 960mg, Potassium 20%, Total Carbohydrates 8g, Dietary Fiber 3g, Sugars 6g, Protein 3g, Vitamin A 10%, Vitamin C 80%, Calcium 4%

Savory baked acorn squash

This is a savory dish. For the classic sweet version, leave out the pepper and swap some brown sugar, butter, and cinnamon for the Paremesan, olive oil, and paprika.

Prep time: 5 minutes
Cook time: 30 minutes
Total time: 35 minutes

Ingredients
1 acorn squash
kosher salt and fresh ground pepper
freshly grated Parmesan cheese, optional
2 tsp. olive oil
smoked paprika

Instructions
1. Ensure your oven is heated to 425 degrees Fahrenheit.
2. Cut acorn squash in half lengthwise, then cut halves into quarters lengthwise. Scoop out seeds and discard.
3. Place the squash on baking sheet and drizzle olive oil over top of each quarter. Scatter with the smoked paprika, salt and pepper and bake in oven for 30 minutes.
4. Garnish with the Parmesan if desired.

Nutrition Facts Serves: 4
Calories 80, Fat Calories 25, Total Fat 25g, Saturated Fat 0 g, Cholesterol 0 mg, Sodium 200mg, Trans Fat 0 g, Potassium 13%, Total Carbohydrates 14g, Dietary Fiber 3 g, Sugars 0g, Protein 3 g, Vitamin A 35%, Vitamin C 25%, Calcium 6%, Iron 15%

Roasted Brussels sprouts

If you've never had crispy, caramelized Brussels sprouts, you need to try these. The taste and texture both hold up extremely well in the fridge.

Prep time: 5 minutes
Cook time: 15 minutes
Total time: 20 minutes

Ingredients
1/4 tsp. sea salt
1/4 tsp. ground black pepper
3/4 pounds Brussel sprouts, sliced in half length-wise
1 1/2 T. melted ghee

Instructions
1. Ensure your oven is heated to 400 degrees Fahrenheit. Cut Brussels sprouts in half and place in a medium sized bowl. Drizzle the olive oil over the Brussels sprouts and then toss with the sea salt and black pepper until evenly coated.
2. Pour Brussels sprouts onto a baking sheet and make sure they are evenly spaced so that they will roast easily.
3. Place the sheet in the oven and let it cook approximately 10 minutes before stirring well and returning it to the oven for 10 minutes more. Season with pepper and salt as needed They will keep in the fridge for 3-4 days, or in the freezer for 2-3 months.

Nutrition Facts Serves: 4
Calories 60, Calories From Fat 45, Total Fat 5g, Saturated Fat 5g, Trans Fat 0g, Cholesterol 0mg, Sodium 200mg, Potassium 4%, Total Carbohydrates 4g, Dietary Fiber 2g, Sugars 1g, Protein 1g 2%, Vitamin A 4%, Vitamin C 35%, Calcium 2%, Iron 6%

Roasted rosemary potatoes

It's hard to imagine a protein that wouldn't go well with this side.

Prep time: 10 minutes
Cook time: 25 minutes
Total time: 35 minutes

Ingredients
1 head of garlic
3 sprigs of rosemary
3 sprigs of thyme
20 oz. baby potatoes
2 T parsley, chopped
Sea salt, to taste
Ground black pepper, to taste
2 T olive oil

Instructions
1. Ensure your oven is heated to 450 degrees Fahrenheit.
2. Separate garlic cloves and remove the papery skin holding them together, but do not peel.
3. Add the rosemary, thyme, baby potatoes, parsley, garlic and olive oil together in a large bowl, coating well.
4. Add the results to a jelly roll pan that has been lined with tinfoil before topping with pepper and salt. Place the pan in the oven and let the potatoes bake approximately 25 minutes, stirring at the 12-minute mark.
5. Season with additional pepper and salt prior to serving.

Nutrition Facts Serves: 6
Calories 151, Sodium 101 mg, Total Fat 7 g, Potassium 483 mg, Saturated Fat 1 g, Carbs 20 g, Protein 2 g, Polyunsaturated Fat 3 g, Monounsaturated Fat 2 g, Sugars 1 g, Trans Fat 0 g, Dietary Fiber 3 g, Calcium 1%, Vitamin C 30%, Iron 5%

Bean and beef enchiladas

This recipe, along with the chicken enchilada recipe, is great as a frozen meal. Just double the recipe, and prepare one in a foil pan. Don't cook it, but instead wrap it in plastic and then foil, and freeze for 2-3 months. The plastic will keep it fresh, but it's probably worth writing a reminder to yourself to take off the plastic when you reheat it. Reheat in a 350 degree oven for 50 minutes, covered with the foil. Take the foil off during the last ten minutes of cooking.

Prep time: 30 minutes
Cook time: 30 minutes
Total time: 1 hour

Ingredients
3 ½ cups of water
1 T lime juice
½ cups of chicken broth, low sodium, fat free
2/3 cups of black beans, drained and rinsed
1 T tomato paste, low-sodium
Kosher sea salt, to taste
½ tsp. cumin, ground
6 T crema, Mexican style
3 onions, divided, sliced
2 oz. shredded Monterey Jack
2 ½ oz. shredded cheddar cheese
12 corn tortillas
1 tsp. oregano, Mexican variety
4 tsp. garlic, minced
2 cups of onion, chopped
2 tsp. olive oil
8 oz. sirloin, ground
28 oz. can enchilada sauce (red or green)

Equipment
13x9" dish

Instructions

1. Preheat oven to 400 degrees Fahrenheit.
2. Place a skillet on top of a stove over a burner set to a high/medium heat before adding in the beef and letting it brown for 5 minutes. Remove it from the pan and let it drain.
3. Wipe out the pan and return pan to medium heat. Place more oil in the pan; swirl to coat. Add onion; cook until tender, stir as needed
4. Add garlic, oregano, cumin and salt and let it cook 2 minutes while still stirring before adding in the tomato paste and letting everything cook an additional minute.
5. Add in the broth, beans and beef and let everything cook another minute, still stirring. After you have removed it from heat, add in the lime juice.
6. Wrap six tortillas at a time in a wet paper towel covering the top and the bottom. Microwave for 45 seconds or until soft. In each tortilla, at 3 T of the beef before rolling tightly.
7. Add half a cup of the sauce to the bottom of a glass baking dish (13 x 9) that has been prepared using cooking spray before placing the enchiladas into the dish. Pour remaining enchilada sauce over the enchiladas. Top with the cheeses.
8. Add the dish to the oven and let it bake at 400 degrees Fahrenheit approximately 20 minutes. You are looking for it to be lightly browned and bubbly. Let the enchiladas stand 10 minutes. Top with the green onions and crema if serving immediately. This makes a great frozen dish.

Nutrition Facts Serves: 4

Calories 343, Fat 15.4 g, Saturated fat 5.8 g, Monounsaturated fat 5.1 g, Polyunsaturated fat 1.4 g, Carbohydrate 35 g, Cholesterol 50 mg, Sodium 540 mg, Calcium 236 mg, Protein 18.5 g, Fiber 7 g, Iron 1.6 mg.

Fast and tasty chicken enchiladas

This can quickly and easily be turned into a vegetarian dish by adding either pinto beans or black beans in place of the chicken.

Prep time: 20 mins
Cook time: 46 mins
Total time: 66 mins

Ingredients
2 cups of Monterey cheese, shredded
19 oz. premade enchilada sauce
2 large chicken breasts
6, 6-inch tortillas

Equipment
Baking dish

Instructions
1. Portion each breast into 3 pieces to allow it to cook more quickly before adding it to a pot and topping with enchilada sauce.
2. Place the pot onto the stove on top of a burner set to a medium/low heat and let the chicken simmer for 20 minutes until it is cooked. Take care to stir regularly to prevent it from sticking.
3. Turn your oven to 375 degrees Fahrenheit and shred the chicken using a pair of forks.
4. Add ¼ cup of enchilada sauce to the bottom of a baking dish before adding in a pair of tortillas, 1/3 the total chicken and 1/3 the sauce from the pot and 1/3 of the cheese. Create two more layers comprised of sauce, tortillas, chicken, chicken sauce and cheese.

5. Place the dish into the oven and let it cook for 25 minutes.
6. Portion the casserole out into individual containers and keep in fridge for 3-4 days. Alternatively, wrap with plastic wrap and foil and freeze for 2-3 months.

<u>Nutrition Facts</u> Serves: 6

Calories 330, Calories From Fat 170, Total Fat 18g, Saturated Fat 11g, Trans Fat 0g, Cholesterol 75mg, Sodium 930mg, Potassium 7%, Total Carbohydrates 17g, Dietary Fiber 3g, Sugars 5g, Protein 24g, Vitamin A 20%, Vitamin C 4%, Calcium45%, Iron8%

Sweet potato wedges

These potato wedges are better than French fries in every way imaginable. Spoiler alert: you can use the same technique with potatoes as well. Just check every 10 minutes to make sure they don't get overdone. Another variation would be to sprinkle over a little grated Parmesan in the last ten minutes of cooking.

Prep time: 10 minutes
Cook time: 30 minutes
Total time: 40 minutes

Ingredients
1 tsp. salt
1 tsp. cracked black pepper
1/2 tsp. garlic powder
4 medium peeled sweet potatoes (about 2 1/2 pounds), each cut into 6 wedges
1 T chopped fresh rosemary
2 T olive oil

Instructions
1. Preheat oven to 450 degrees Fahrenheit.
2. In a mixing bowl, combine the olive oil, rosemary, sweet potatoes, garlic powder, black pepper and salt together and ensure the potatoes are coated well.
3. Add the results in a single layer to a large roasting pan before placing the pan in the oven and letting the potatoes bake for 20 minutes. Turn the dish at this point before baking another 10 minutes.

Nutrition Facts Serves: 6
Calories 129, Fat 4.5 g, Saturated fat 0.6 g, Protein 1.4 g, Carbohydrate 22.5 g, Cholesterol 0 mg, Iron 0.3 mg, Sodium 418 mg, Calories from fat 31 %, Fiber 2.8 g, Calcium 16 mg

Slow cooker pulled pork shoulder

If you're a fan of barbecue, this might become your favorite dish. It uses a cheap cut of meat and can be customized with the barbecue sauce of your choosing.

Prep time: 10 minutes
Cook time: 5 hours
Total time: 5 hours 10 minutes

Ingredients
2 tsp. ground black pepper
1 onion, roughly chopped
4 cloves garlic, finely minced or pressed through a garlic press
1/2 cup dry white wine (or use chicken broth)
1 3 -to-4-pound boneless pork shoulder (or 4 1/2-pound bone-in pork shoulder)
1 T kosher salt

Instructions
1. Rinse the pork, place on a cutting board, trim off any excess fat, pat dry with paper towels and rub in the salt and pepper. Add the pork to the slow cooker, scatter the onion on top of the pork, sprinkle in the garlic as well as the wine. Cook for 5 hours or until the meat can be easily shredded with use of a knife.
2. Turn off the slow cooker and remove the pork to a platter. Shred the meat with two forks.

Nutrition Facts Serves: 8 (6 oz. serving)
Calories 195, Protein 20 g, Total Fat 12 g

Best lentil curry

The combination of fresh ginger and garlic along with the curry powder is what makes this an exceptional, yet simple dish.

Prep time: 10 min
Cook time: 30 minutes
Total time: 40 minutes

Ingredients
4 cups of vegetable broth, low sodium
1 cup of lentils, red
10 oz. potato, peeled and made into pieces that are 1 inch each
8 oz. of carrot, chopped
Curry powder, 1 T
8 scallions, separated, sliced
2 garlic cloves chopped
2 T chopped ginger
3 T canola oil

Instructions
1. Add the oil to a saucepan before placing it on the stove on top of a burner set to a high/medium heat.
2. Add in the scallion whites, garlic and ginger and let them soften for 2 minutes.
3. Mix in the curry powder as well as pepper and salt, to taste, broth, lentils, potato and carrots before letting everything boil. Turn down the heat and let everything simmer for 15 minutes, stirring regularly.
4. Top with scallion greens prior to serving.

Nutrition Facts Serves: 4
Calories 374, calcium 77 mg, iron, 3 mg, fiber 6 g, sugar 6 g, carbohydrates 45 g, protein, 20 g, sodium 550 mg, cholesterol 6 mg, saturated fat 1 g, fat 11 g

Chana masala

This recipe is easily doubled or tripled. The only limitation is the size of your pot.

Prep time: 5 minutes
Cook time: 25 minutes
Total time: 30 minutes

Ingredients
1 tsp. curry powder
32 oz. chickpeas, rinsed, drained
2 cloves of garlic, minced
1 large onion, chopped
1 T extra virgin olive oil
¼ cups of cilantro
Kosher sea salt, to taste
1 T lemon juice
2 tomatoes, chopped
2 tsp. ginger, grated
½ tsp. turmeric

Instructions
1. Add the oil to a skillet before placing it on a burner set to a medium/high heat. Add in the onion and let it sauté until it has become translucent and soft. Mix in the garlic and let it cook for 3 minutes.
2. Add in the curry powder, chickpeas, olive oil, lemon juice, tomatoes, ginger and turmeric along with ¼ cups of water. Let the mixture simmer before cooking it for 10 minutes, stirring on occasion. The end result should have a stew like consistency but not be runny.
3. Season using salt and top with cilantro prior to serving.

Nutrition Facts Serves: 4
330 Calories, 14 g Protein, 7 g Fiber, 5 g, Total Fat, 46 g Carbohydrates, 672 mg Sodium

Oven farro risotto

Again, make sure to get the perlato farro. This recipe is an improvement on stove-top risotto made with rice. It is higher in protein and lower in fat than those traditional recipes.

Prep time: 10 minutes
Cook time: 45 minutes
Total time: 1 hour

Ingredients
2 T olive oil, plus more to grease the baking pan and for drizzling
zest of one lemon
1 medium onion
Salt, to taste
1 cup freshly grated Parmesan
1 T fresh oregano, chopped
1 1/2 cups uncooked perlato farro
1 cup / 8 oz tomato sauce*
2 1/2 cups vegetable broth or water

Equipment
8x8 inch baking dish

Instructions

1. Preheat oven to 400 degrees. Place the rack in the top third of the oven. Rub the olive oil on the bottom and sides of the 8x8-inch baking dish and sprinkle with the lemon zest.

2. Place a saucepan on the stove on top of a burner set to a high/medium heat. Combine the olive oil, onion, and a pinch of salt. Cook until the onions soften and become translucent, 3-5 minutes. Add the farro and stir until thoroughly moistened, and cook for 1-2 minutes. Stir in the tomato sauce and the broth, then bring to a simmer, but not boiling. Remove from heat, and stir in about one cup of the cheese.

3. Pour into the baking dish, cover with foil, poke a few slits in the foil, and bake the mixture for about 45 minutes or until fully cooked. The farro should be al dente, not totally soft but with a little resistance to it. You can uncover in the last few minutes to brown the risotto. You may also choose to finish it under the broiler for 3-4 minutes. Sprinkle with the remaining cheese, the fresh oregano, and top with olive oil to serve. It can be kept in the fridge for 3-4 days or in the freezer for 2-3 months

Nutrition Facts: Serves: 6, Calories: 110, Total Fat 7g, Saturated Fat 25g, Trans Fat 0g, Cholesterol 10mg, Sodium 1000mg, Potassium 6%, Total Carbohydrates 7g, Dietary Fiber 2g, Sugars 3g, Protein 5g, Vitamin A10%, Vitamin C 30%, Calcium 15%, Iron 6%

Basic oven brown rice

This is the easiest way to cook a large volume of rice, unless you have an extra-large rice cooker. Rice freezes well.

Prep time: 5 minutes
Cook time: 1 hour
Total time: 1 hour 15 minutes

Ingredients
1/4 tsp. kosher salt
3 cups long grain brown rice
5 cups water
1 T olive oil

Equipment
6-quart Dutch oven or other heavy-bottomed pot with lid

Instructions
1. Ensure your oven is set at 375 degrees.
2. In a 6-quart Dutch oven or heavy bottomed pot on the stove, heat water, oil and salt until boiling. Stir in rice, remove from stove, cover pot and place in the hot oven.
3. Bake for 1 hour without stirring.
4. Remove from oven, remove lid and fluff with a fork.
5. This recipe makes 9 cups rice.

<u>Nutrition Facts</u> Serves: 9
Calories 216, Sodium 10 mg, Potassium 84 mg, Carbohydrates 45 g, Polyunsaturated 1 g, Monounsaturated 1 g, Sugars 1 g, Protein 5 g, Calcium 2%, Iron 5%, Total Fat 3 g, Dietary Fiber 3 g.

Chapter 9: Snacks

Customizable maple granola

Use all your favorite ingredients to make this granola your own.

Prep time: 5 minutes
Cook time: 23 minutes
Total time: 28 minutes

Ingredients
4 cups old-fashioned rolled oats
1½ cup raw nuts and/or seeds
1 tsp. fine-grain sea salt ½ tsp. cinnamon
½ cup melted coconut oil or olive oil
½ cup maple syrup or honey
1 tsp. vanilla extract
⅔ cup dried fruit

Instructions
1. Preheat oven to 350 degree. Line a large, rimmed baking sheet with a sheet of parchment paper. In a large mixing bowl, stir together the oats, nuts and/or seeds, salt and cinnamon.
2. Add the oil, maple syrup and/or honey and vanilla. Mix well, until thoroughly coated. Pour the granola onto your prepared pan and spread it in an even layer with a large spoon. Bake until golden, about 21 to 23 minutes, stirring halfway through cooking time.
3. Cool granola completely before breaking it into pieces and stirring in the dried fruit. The granola can be stored in an airtight container at room temperature for 1 to 2 weeks, or in a sealed freezer bag in the freezer for up to 3 months.

Nutrition Facts Serves: 12
Calories 98, Total Fat 2 g, Total Carbs 2g, Protein 20 g

Healthier dark chocolate almond butter cups

These are the adult version of that other candy and a healthier choice to treat yourself after a long day of meal prep.

Ingredients
Kosher salt, as garnish
¼ tsp. sea salt
¼ cups agave syrup
2 T melted coconut oil
½ cups almond butter
12 oz. semisweet chocolate, chopped fine

Equipment
Muffin pan
Muffin liners
Pastry brush (optional)

Instructions

1. Prepare a muffin tray by lining it with plastic liners.
2. Place the chocolate into a small pan before placing the pan on top of the stove over a burner set to a low heat and stir while it melts.
3. After the chocolate, has melted most of the way, remove the pan from heat and keep stirring until the remainder has melted.
4. Add 1 ½ tsp. of chocolate to each muffin liner and ensure it covers have an inch of space. The chocolate should be as even as possible before you place it in the refrigerator to cool for 15 minutes or until it has solidified.
5. While the chocolate cools, take a small bowl and add in the salt, agave syrup, coconut oil and almond butter and mix well, the results should be completely smooth which may require the use of a small pastry brush.
6. Add the results to the top of the chocolate in the lined muffin tin and smooth it out as best as you can before adding an extra 1 tsp. of chocolate to the top of each cup.
7. Top with sea salt and let them refrigerate an additional 30 minutes to ensure they harden properly.
8. These will keep in the refrigerator for up to three weeks as long as they are held in a container that is completely air tight.

Nutrition Facts Serves: 12

Calories: 238, Total Fat: 18 g, Saturated Fat: 7 g, Carbohydrates: 21 g, Fiber: 4 g, Sugars: 13.5 g, Protein: 3 g, Sodium: 242 mg, Cholesterol: 0 mg, Monounsaturated Fat: 7 g.

Chili lime pumpkin seeds

This snack is great whether eaten by the handful or sprinkled on a simple green salad.

Ingredients
1 1/2 T lime juice
1/3 tsp. cayenne pepper
1/4 tsp. sea salt
zest of half a lime
2 cups pumpkin seeds
1 T chili powder
2 T extra virgin olive oil

Instructions
1. Preheat oven to 350 degrees Fahrenheit.
2. Mix together olive oil, lime juice and pumpkin seeds in a small bowl.
3. Mix in chili powder, cayenne pepper, and salt. Stir to coat.
4. Spread the seeds onto a baking sheet lined with foil in an even layer. Bake for half an houre. Stir the seeds halfway through.
5. Cool before adding lime zest. Add salt to taste.
6. To store, place in a container that is air tight at room temperature for 1 or 2 weeks, or in a sealed freezer bag in the freezer for up to 3 months.

Nutrition Facts Serves: 4
Calories 30, Fat based calories 8, Total Fat 2 g, Trans Fat 0 g, Sodium 100mg, Potassium 2%, Total Carbohydrates 5g, Protein 1 g, Dietary Fiber 3 g, Vitamin A 16%, Vitamin C 15%, Calcium 4%, Iron 6%, Saturated Fat 0 g, Cholesterol 0 mg, Sugars 1 g.

Conclusion

Thank for making it through to the end of *Meal Prep: The Practical Guide to Preparing Quick Delicious Meals for Weight Loss, No Stress, And Faster Fat-Burning Results*. Let's hope it was informative and able to provide you with all of the tools you need to achieve your goals whatever they may be.

The next step is to experiment with your meal prep. Try different cooking and storage techniques. Also test new seasonings, meat, grains and produce. Plan your meals, but be creative!

Finally, if you found this book useful in any way, a review on Amazon is always appreciated!